# Faqs of Cosmetic Surgery: A Guide for Patients

Daniel Gallaga, MD

# Faqs of Cosmetic Surgery: A Guide for Patients

Daniel Gallaga, MD

Copyright © 2024 **Daniel Gallaga.**

All rights reserved. No part of this book may be reproduced by any mechanical, photographic, or electronic process or in the form of phonographic recording, scanning, or otherwise, except as permitted by the Mexican Copyright Act, without prior written permission of the author

# Welcome

Hello! I'm Dr. Daniel Gallaga.

Welcome to this no-nonsense guide to cosmetic surgery. If you're considering getting a little work done, you're in the right place! Here, I'll tell you everything you need to know to make your best decision.

# Table of Contents

Chapter 1 ........................................................................................... 11
  What's the Deal with Cosmetic Surgery? ................................... 11
    The Dilemma of Self-Esteem vs. Vanity ................................ 12
    Cosmetic Surgery as a Tool for Transformation ................... 13

Chapter 2 ........................................................................................... 15
  Breast Augmentation: Everything You Need to Know to Boost Your Confidence ................................................................. 15
    What is Breast Augmentation Surgery? ................................ 15
    Am I a Good Candidate for Breast Augmentation? ............. 15
    What Types of Implants are There? ...................................... 16
    What is the Surgery Like? ....................................................... 16
    What about Recovery? ............................................................. 17
    What Could go Wrong? ........................................................... 17
    What Size Should I Get? .......................................................... 19
    Other Questions about Breast Surgeries ............................... 20

Chapter 3 ........................................................................................... 21
  Blepharoplasty: Rejuvenate Your Look! ..................................... 21
    What is Blepharoplasty, and Who is it for? .......................... 21
    How will I Look after Blepharoplasty? ................................. 21
    What is the Surgery and Recovery Like? .............................. 22
    What Risks Should I Consider? .............................................. 22
    Frequently Asked Questions about Blepharoplasty ............. 22

Chapter 4 ........................................................................................... 25
  Liposuction: A Complete Guide .................................................. 25
    What is Liposuction? ............................................................... 25
    Fat Transfer to the Buttocks (BBL) ......................................... 27

Ultrasound-guided BBL ........................................................ 28

## Chapter 5 ........................................................................... 31

### Nose Surgery: Breathe and Look Better! ............................ 31

What is Nose Surgery? ......................................................... 31

Am I a Good Candidate for Nose Surgery? ......................... 31

What is the Surgery Like? .................................................... 31

What is the Recovery Like? ................................................. 32

What are the Risks? ............................................................. 32

Frequently Asked Questions about Nose Surgery ............... 33

## Chapter 6 ........................................................................... 35

### Tummy Tuck: Get Your Figure Back! ................................. 35

What is a Tummy Tuck? ...................................................... 35

Am I a Good Candidate for a Tummy Tuck? ....................... 35

What Types of Tummy Tucks are There? ............................ 35

What is the Surgery Like? .................................................... 36

What is the Recovery Like? ................................................. 36

What are the Risks? ............................................................. 36

Frequently Asked Questions about Tummy Tucks .............. 37

## Chapter 7 ........................................................................... 39

### Facial and Neck Rejuvenation: Refresh Your Face! .............. 39

What is Facial and Neck Rejuvenation? ............................... 39

Am I a Good Candidate for this Type of Surgery? ............... 39

What Types of Rejuvenation are There? ............................... 39

What is the Surgery Like? .................................................... 40

What is the Recovery Like? ................................................. 40

What are the Risks? ............................................................. 41

Frequently Asked Questions about Facial and Neck
Rejuvenation ........................................................................ 42

Chapter 8 ............................................................................................... 45
   Intimate Surgery: Regain Your Confidence and Well-being!.. 45
      What is Intimate Surgery? ........................................................ 45
      Am I a Good Candidate for Intimate Surgery? ...................... 45
      Types of Intimate Surgery ........................................................ 45
      What are the Operations Like? ................................................ 46
      What is Recovery Like?............................................................. 46
      What Risks are There?............................................................... 47
      Frequently Asked Questions about Intimate Surgery .......... 47
Chapter 9 ............................................................................................... 49
   Other Cosmetic Surgeries and Treatments: Explore your options! ................................................................................................. 49
      What other Cosmetic Surgeries are There? ............................ 49
      What Non-surgical Treatments exist?..................................... 49
Chapter 10 ............................................................................................. 51
   Pre- and Post-Operative Care: Get Ready to Look Amazing!. 51
About the Author................................................................................. 55

x

# Chapter 1

## What's the Deal with Cosmetic Surgery?

Cosmetic surgery is like real-life Photoshop, but in 3D. It's used to improve your appearance and make you feel more comfortable with yourself. But remember, it's not magic. With a good surgeon and realistic expectations, the results can be incredible.

Before you start reading this book, it's very important to know that...

- **These procedures are not urgent or necessary.** Cosmetic surgery is a personal decision and should not be taken lightly. Take your time to think about whether it's really what you want and need.
- **During the consultation, I repeatedly say, "You don't need anything I do. What do you want and what are you looking for? My goal is to help you achieve the image you want, giving you the best tools to make your best decision."** A good surgeon will listen to you, advise you, and help you make the best decision for yourself, but the final decision will always be yours.
- **Surgery should flow; it's a stressful situation on its own, and external factors can make it more complex than it already is.** It's important that you feel comfortable and confident with your surgeon and that communication is fluid to avoid misunderstandings and surprises.
- **It's your body, your decision. In the world of good and evil, although there are beauty standards, what you like doesn't necessarily have to be what your

doctor likes. It's important to have a stable doctor-patient relationship and communication so there are no misunderstandings. Your tastes and preferences are important, but so is your surgeon's opinion. Together, you can find the perfect balance to achieve the results you want.
- **The only complication without a solution is death. Most adverse events in cosmetic surgery can be solved or reversed. It usually takes a lot of patience from both the doctor and the patient.** While cosmetic surgery is generally safe, it's important to be aware of the possible risks and complications. A good surgeon will inform you about them and give you the tools to minimize them.

**"Don't Do Anything, You Look Fine As You Are"**

Does this phrase sound familiar? You've probably heard it before, whether from a friend, family member, or even yourself. The topic of cosmetic surgery always generates mixed opinions. While some people see it as a tool to improve their self-esteem and feel more confident, others consider it unnecessary and even dangerous.

But what's the truth? Is cosmetic surgery only for the vain, or can it really help improve our self-esteem?

## The Dilemma of Self-Esteem vs. Vanity

Self-esteem is the appreciation and consideration we have for ourselves. It's fundamental to our emotional well-being and our ability to relate with others. Vanity, on the other hand, is excessive pride in our own merits and the desire to be admired and recognized for them.

In the context of cosmetic surgery, it's important to distinguish between seeking to improve our appearance out of self-love and doing it out of a desire for external approval. The first option can be a valid path to increase our self-esteem and feel more comfortable in our own skin. The second, however, can become an endless pursuit of perfection, driven by insecurity and fear of rejection.

## Cosmetic Surgery as a Tool for Transformation

Many patients who seek cosmetic surgery don't do it out of vanity, but out of a genuine desire to improve aspects of their appearance that cause them insecurity or discomfort. Phrases like "Doctor, I don't want to look so angry" or "I look in the mirror and it's not me" are common in cosmetic surgery consultations.

Cosmetic surgery can be a powerful tool to transform our appearance and, with it, our perception of ourselves. Studies have shown that improving physical appearance can have a positive impact on people's self-esteem, confidence, and quality of life.

## Conclusion

Cosmetic surgery can be a powerful tool to improve our self-esteem and make us feel more comfortable in our own skin. However, it's important to do it for the right reasons and with the guidance of a qualified and ethical plastic surgeon.

Remember, beauty is not just about physical appearance, but also about how we feel about ourselves. Love yourself, take care of yourself, and make the best decisions for you!

# Bibliography

- American Society of Plastic Surgeons. (2023). What is plastic surgery? https://www.plasticsurgery.org/
- Mayo Clinic. (2023). Cosmetic surgery. https://www.mayoclinic.org/tests-procedures/cosmetic-surgery/about/pac-20385138
- Veale, D. (2004). Body dysmorphic disorder. American Journal of Psychiatry, 161(5), 766-777.
- Phillips, K. A. (2005). The broken mirror: Understanding and treating body dysmorphic disorder. Oxford University Press.

# Chapter 2

## Breast Augmentation: Everything You Need to Know to Boost Your Confidence

Have you looked in the mirror and wished you had larger, lifted, or more symmetrical breasts? You're not alone! Many women seek to improve the appearance of their breasts to feel more confident and comfortable with their bodies. In this chapter, we'll discuss everything you need to know about breast augmentation surgery, also known as augmentation mammoplasty.

### What is Breast Augmentation Surgery?

Breast augmentation surgery is a surgical procedure that aims to increase the size and improve the shape of your breasts. This is achieved by placing breast implants, which are prostheses filled with saline solution or silicone gel inside the breast.

### Am I a Good Candidate for Breast Augmentation?

Breast augmentation surgery may be an excellent option for you if:

- You want to increase the size of your breasts.
- You want to improve the shape and symmetry of your breasts.
- You have lost volume in your breasts after pregnancy or breastfeeding.
- You feel uncomfortable with the size or shape of your breasts.

However, it's important to have realistic expectations and understand that surgery is not a magic solution for all self-esteem issues. Ideally, you should be in good physical and mental health and have a clear idea of the results you expect to achieve.

## What Types of Implants are There?

There are two main types of breast implants:

- **Saline implants:** These are filled with sterile salt water and can be adjusted in size during surgery.
- **Silicone gel implants:** These are filled with a cohesive silicone gel and offer a more natural feel.

The choice of implant type will depend on your personal preferences, your anatomy, and the recommendations of your plastic surgeon.

## What is the Surgery Like?

Breast augmentation surgery is performed under combined anesthesia epidural with sedation and usually lasts between 1 and 2 hours. The cosmetic surgeon will make an incision in one of these three areas:

- Inframammary fold: below the breast.
- Areola: around the nipple.
- Axilla: in the armpit.

Through this incision, the surgeon will create a pocket to place the implant, either under or over the pectoral muscle. Then, they will close the incision with sutures.

## What about Recovery?

Recovery from breast augmentation surgery varies from person to person, but in general, you can expect:

- **Swelling and bruising:** This is normal and will gradually disappear in the weeks following surgery.
- **Mild discomfort:** You may feel some pain, but it can be controlled with medication.
- **Wearing a special bra:** This will help support and protect your breasts during recovery.
- **Rest and avoid strenuous activities:** It's important to rest and avoid lifting heavy objects during the first few weeks.

Most women can return to normal activities in 1-2 weeks, but following your plastic surgeon's instructions is important for optimal recovery.

## What Could go Wrong?

Like any surgery, breast augmentation surgery has certain risks, such as:

- **Infection:** (less than 1% of cases)
- **Bleeding:** (less than 2% of cases)
- **Reactions to anesthesia:** (varies depending on the type of anesthesia and the patient's health)
- **Scars:** (although plastic surgeons try to make them as discreet as possible, there will always be scars)
- **Capsular contracture:** (5-10% of cases)
- **Implant rupture:** (1-2% of cases in the first 10 years)

It's important to talk to your plastic surgeon about all the possible risks and complications before making a decision.

In 2018, studies were conducted in Europe that showed textured implants, on average after 10 years in populations with certain factors, cause CANCER. The intention is to inform, not to generate hysteria or panic. "Doctor, I have implants. Do I have cancer?" The answer would be NO, it's only a specific type of implant. The incidence in other countries is relatively low, but it is a risk. If the patient is healthy, why put their health at risk? Ignorance would be the biggest sin of omission in this particular case, falling into negligence.

If textured implants (those linked to causing cancer) are knowingly used, it's serious and unethical. Plastic surgeons continue to use them because "commercial" houses continue to sell them. Health is not a commodity. There has been a "recall" in the EC (European Commission) of textured implants as they are directly linked to GIANT CELL CANCER (BIA-ALCL breast implant-associated anaplastic large cell lymphoma).

In cases where breast augmentation or reconstruction surgery has already been performed and the type of implant used is unknown, the clinical practice guidelines (2019) recommend:

- **Step 1:** Ultrasound. If findings or data are present, proceed to the next step. An ultrasound-guided aspiration can be performed to take samples.
- **Step 2:** Magnetic Resonance Imaging (MRI). If there is suspicion, preservation of breast tissue will be recommended.
- **Step 3:** Fine needle aspiration. Certain tumor markers are sought. If positive, surgery is recommended.

- **Step 4:** Conservative surgery. Depending on the stage, radiotherapy or chemotherapy, as well as co-adjuvant treatments, will be important to consider.

It's important to clarify that there is no restriction in Mexico on the sale of textured implants. There has been evidence of bribes to medical groups to downplay the situation. Certain brands have taken it upon themselves to suspend the manufacture and sale of these implants. Smooth, round implants in a sub-facial or sub-muscular plane are recommended for aesthetic purposes.

## What Size Should I Get?

This is one of the most frequent questions my patients ask me. We usually talk about bra sizes, and some patients have an idea, but even the size varies from brand to brand. It's your body and your decision, although I'm more inclined towards smaller or more conservative implants.

The truth is, there's no single answer for everyone. The ideal implant size will depend on your personal preferences, your anatomy, and your lifestyle.

In the consultation, what we want to visualize is how much they would grow, and I explain it to them with 3 different sizes. Assuming you're 5'5" and have a slim build (A cup), a 380cc silicone gel implant would be my recommendation. Anything above that size can be more eye-catching, without being vulgar, and anything smaller would be more conservative.

The exercise in the consultation is how "operated" you want to look. All answers are correct. There are patients who just want to fill in "gaps," others who want a good cleavage that attracts attention when wearing a tight red dress, and the middle ground is patients who want it to "be noticeable but not too noticeable, but still see the change."

## Other Questions about Breast Surgeries

- **How long do implants last?** Breast implants don't have a specific lifespan, but it's recommended to replace them every 10-15 years.
- **Will I be able to breastfeed after surgery?** In most cases, breast augmentation surgery doesn't affect breastfeeding ability.
- **Does breast augmentation surgery cause breast cancer?** There is no scientific evidence that breast augmentation surgery causes breast cancer.

**Bibliography**

- American Society of Plastic Surgeons. (2023). Breast Augmentation. https://www.plasticsurgery.org/cosmetic-procedures/breast-augmentation
- Mayo Clinic. (2023). Breast augmentation. https://www.mayoclinic.org/tests-procedures/breast-augmentation/doctors-departments/pdc-20393180

# Chapter 3

## Blepharoplasty: Rejuvenate Your Look!

Do your eyes betray you and make you look more tired than you feel? Blepharoplasty might be the solution! This surgery helps remove excess skin, fat, and bags from your eyelids, giving you a fresher, more youthful and rested appearance.

### What is Blepharoplasty, and Who is it for?

Blepharoplasty is a surgical procedure that improves the appearance of your eyelids, both upper and lower. It helps you look younger and corrects functional problems like difficulty seeing due to excess skin.

This surgery is ideal for you if:

- You have droopy or puffy eyelids.
- You notice bags under your eyes.
- You feel your eyes look tired or aged.
- You experience difficulty seeing due to excess skin on your eyelids.

### How will I Look after Blepharoplasty?

After surgery, your eyes will look more open, brighter, and rejuvenated. Blepharoplasty can achieve the following for you:

- Remove excess skin and fat from the eyelids.
- Reduce bags and dark circles.
- Improve the symmetry of your eyes.
- Lift droopy eyelids.

## What is the Surgery and Recovery Like?

Blepharoplasty is performed under local anesthesia with sedation or general anesthesia. The cosmetic surgeon will make discreet incisions in the natural folds of your eyelids to minimize visible scars. Recovery varies, but generally involves:

- Swelling and bruising that gradually disappear.
- Mild discomfort that can be controlled with medication.
- Use of cold compresses to reduce inflammation.
- Avoid strenuous activities during the first few weeks.

## What Risks Should I Consider?

Like any surgery, blepharoplasty carries risks, although they are uncommon. Some of them include:

- Infection: (less than 1% of cases)
- Bleeding: (less than 2% of cases)
- Reactions to anesthesia: (varies depending on the type of anesthesia and the patient's health)
- Temporary blurred vision: (less than 5% of cases)
- Asymmetry in the eyelids: (less than 3% of cases)
- Dry eye: (5-15% of cases)

## Frequently Asked Questions about Blepharoplasty

- **How long do the results last?** The results can last many years, although natural aging will continue. On average, it can be summarized as 5 to 10 years.
- **When can I return to my activities?** Most people return to their activities in 1-2 weeks.

- **Will there be visible scars?** The scars are usually minimal and hidden in the natural folds of the eyelids.

**Bibliography**

- American Society of Plastic Surgeons. (2023). Eyelid surgery. https://www.plasticsurgery.org/cosmetic-procedures/eyelid-surgery
- Kakizaki, H., Malhotra, R., Madge, S. N., & Selva, D. (2017). Upper Eyelid Blepharoplasty. In Plastic Surgery (pp. 311-324). Springer, Cham.
- Codner, M. A., McCord, C. D., & Codner, E. M. (2018). Eyelid & Periocular Rejuvenation. In Decision Making in Facial Plastic Surgery (pp. 115-144). Elsevier.

*Blepharoplasty*

# Chapter 4

## Liposuction: A Complete Guide

Do you have stubborn areas of fat that just won't budge, no matter how much you diet and exercise? Liposuction might be the answer! This popular cosmetic procedure can help you sculpt your body and achieve a more contoured silhouette.

**What is Liposuction?**

Liposuction is a surgical procedure that removes excess fat deposits from specific areas of your body, such as the abdomen, thighs, arms, neck, or back. It's not a weight loss method but a body sculpting technique to improve your contours.

**Am I a Good Candidate for Liposuction?**

The best candidates for liposuction are:

- **People with stable weight:** Liposuction is not a solution for obesity. It's most effective in people with stable weight who want to eliminate localized areas of fat resistant to diet and exercise.
- **People in good health:** It's important to be in good overall health and not have medical conditions that could increase the risks of surgery.
- **People with realistic expectations:** Liposuction improves body contours but is not a miracle procedure. It's essential to have realistic expectations about the results.

## Liposuction Techniques

There are several liposuction techniques, each with its own advantages:

- **Tumescent liposuction:** This is the most common technique. A tumescent solution (a mixture of local anesthetic, epinephrine, and saline solution) is injected into the treatment area, reducing bleeding and pain.

- **Ultrasound-assisted liposuction (UAL):** This uses ultrasonic energy to break down fat cells, making them easier to remove. It's useful for fibrous areas or areas with thicker skin.

- **Laser-assisted liposuction (LAL):** This uses laser energy to liquefy fat and stimulate collagen production, which can improve skin firmness.

## What can I expect during Liposuction Recovery?

Liposuction recovery varies depending on the extent of the procedure and the technique used. In general, you can expect:

- **Swelling and bruising:** These are common and gradually decrease in the weeks following surgery.
- **Use of compression garments:** These are used to reduce swelling and help the skin adapt to the new contour.
- **Limited physical activity:** It's important to avoid strenuous activities during the first few weeks.
- **Gradual results:** The final results of liposuction are seen as the swelling subsides and the skin retracts.

## Risks and Complications of Liposuction (with percentages)

Although liposuction is generally safe, there are potential risks and complications, such as:

- **Minor complications (5-10%):** Hematomas, seromas (fluid accumulation), contour irregularities, mild infections, etc.
- **Major complications (0.1-1%):** Venous thromboembolism (blood clot formation), pulmonary embolisms, organ perforations, skin necrosis, etc.
- **Mortality (0.002%):** The mortality rate is extremely low.

## Frequently Asked Questions About Liposuction

- **How long does liposuction last?** The duration varies depending on the extent of the procedure, but it can range from 1 to 4 hours.
- **How long do the results last?** The results of liposuction can be long-lasting if you maintain a stable weight and a healthy lifestyle.
- **Does liposuction leave scars?** The incisions are small, and the scars are usually discreet.
- **When can I return to work?** Most people can return to work in 1-2 weeks, depending on the nature of their work.

## Fat Transfer to the Buttocks (BBL)

Fat transfer to the buttocks, also known as a Brazilian Butt Lift (BBL), is a procedure that has gained immense popularity in recent years. It combines liposuction to remove fat from unwanted areas with the injection of that same fat into the buttocks to increase their volume and improve their shape.

## History and Trends

The BBL has its roots in Brazil and has evolved thanks to advances in surgical techniques and technology. Currently, it's one of the fastest-growing cosmetic surgery procedures, driven by the desire to achieve more voluptuous and curvy buttocks.

## Safety Considerations

Safety is a primary concern in BBL. Adverse events related to fat embolism have led to a greater focus on safety protocols, surgical guidelines, and ethical practices. It's crucial for medical professionals to stay informed and prioritize patient well-being.

## Ultrasound-guided BBL

An innovative technique is ultrasound-guided BBL, which uses real-time ultrasound technology to visualize the injection areas and ensure precise fat placement. This can improve the safety of the procedure and minimize the risk of complications like fat embolism.

## Advantages of Ultrasound-guided BBL

- **Greater precision:** Allows for precise fat placement, resulting in more predictable and aesthetically pleasing results.
- **Improved fat viability:** Proper fat placement can improve its long-term survival.

- **Reduced risk of fat embolism:** Real-time visualization helps avoid injecting fat into blood vessels.
- **Faster recovery:** The procedure is less traumatic, which can speed up recovery.

## Disadvantages of Ultrasound-guided BBL

- **Cost:** Ultrasound equipment can increase the cost of the procedure.
- **Learning curve:** Surgeons need specialized training in ultrasound imaging.
- **Time:** The procedure may take longer due to the use of ultrasound.
- **Limited availability:** Not all surgeons offer this technique.

## The Future of BBL

Ultrasound-guided BBL represents a significant advancement in cosmetic surgery. As technology continues to evolve, we'll likely see further improvements in the safety and effectiveness of this procedure.

If you're considering a BBL, it's crucial to discuss all options, including ultrasound-guided BBL, with an experienced cosmetic surgeon.

*Liposuction*

# Chapter 5

## Nose Surgery: Breathe and Look Better!

Have you ever wondered how you would look with a different nose? Nose surgery, or rhinoplasty, is one of the most popular cosmetic procedures and can help you improve both the appearance and function of your nose.

**What is Nose Surgery?**

Rhinoplasty is a surgical procedure that modifies the shape of your nose. It can reduce or increase its size, change the shape of the tip or bridge, narrow the nostrils, or improve the angle between your nose and upper lip. Additionally, it can also correct breathing problems caused by a deviated septum.

**Am I a Good Candidate for Nose Surgery?**

If you're looking to improve the appearance of your nose or correct functional problems, you could be a good candidate! But the most important thing is to have realistic expectations and understand that rhinoplasty won't turn you into someone else. Ideally, you should be in good physical and mental health and have a clear idea of the results you expect to achieve.

**What is the Surgery Like?**

Rhinoplasty is performed under general anesthesia and usually lasts between 1 and 2 hours. The cosmetic surgeon will make incisions inside your nose or on the columella (the skin separating the nostrils) to access the nasal bones and cartilage. Then, they will reshape your nose according to your needs and close the incisions with sutures.

## What is the Recovery Like?

After surgery, it's normal to have some swelling and bruising around your eyes and nose. You might also experience nasal congestion and mild discomfort, which can be controlled with medication. During the first week, you'll need to wear a nasal splint to protect your nose and maintain its new shape. Most people can return to their normal activities in 1-2 weeks, but it's important to follow your cosmetic surgeon's instructions for optimal recovery.

## What are the Risks?

As with any surgery, there are risks associated with rhinoplasty. It's essential to talk to your cosmetic surgeon about all the possible risks and complications before making a decision. Some of the risks include:

- **Infection:** The infection rate after rhinoplasty is low, usually less than 1%.
- **Bleeding:** Excessive bleeding is uncommon, occurring in less than 2% of cases.
- **Scarring problems:** Although the incisions are usually internal, scarring problems can occur in some cases.
- **Adverse reactions to anesthesia:** As with any surgical procedure, there is a small risk of adverse reactions to anesthesia.
- **Need for revision surgery:** In some cases, a second surgery may be necessary to correct details or adjust the results. The percentage of revision surgeries

varies depending on the surgeon and the complexity of the case.
- **Changes in skin sensitivity:** There may be temporary or permanent changes in the sensitivity of the skin on your nose.

## Frequently Asked Questions about Nose Surgery

- **Will it hurt a lot?** Postoperative pain is usually mild and can be controlled with medication.
- **Will I be able to breathe well after surgery?** If the surgery also corrects functional problems, your breathing should improve.
- **How long do the results last?** The results of rhinoplasty are permanent, although natural aging will continue.

## Bibliography

- American Society of Plastic Surgeons. (2023). Rhinoplasty. https://www.plasticsurgery.org/cosmetic-procedures/rhinoplasty
- Rohrich, R. J., & Adams, W. P. Jr. (2001). Rhinoplasty: Art, Science, and New Clinical Techniques.
- Becker, D. G. (2020). Rhinoplasty: An Evidence-Based Approach.

*Nose Surgery*

# Chapter 6

## Tummy Tuck: Get Your Figure Back!

Are you uncomfortable with excess skin or fat on your abdomen? A tummy tuck, or abdominoplasty, can help you regain your figure and feel more confident about your body.

**What is a Tummy Tuck?**

Abdominoplasty is a surgical procedure that removes excess skin and fat from the abdomen and tightens weakened or separated abdominal muscles. This can significantly improve the appearance of your abdomen and give you a more defined silhouette.

**Am I a Good Candidate for a Tummy Tuck?**

If you have excess skin and fat on your abdomen that doesn't respond to diet and exercise, you could be a good candidate! It's also an option if you have weakened or separated abdominal muscles, such as after pregnancy. Ideally, you should be in good physical and mental health and have realistic expectations about the results.

**What Types of Tummy Tucks are There?**

There are different types of abdominoplasty, depending on the extent of the procedure:

- **Full tummy tuck:** Removes excess skin and fat from the entire abdomen and tightens the abdominal muscles.

- **Mini tummy tuck:** Focuses on the lower abdomen and requires a smaller incision.
- **Extended tummy tuck:** Addresses the flanks and lower back in addition to the full tummy tuck.

## What is the Surgery Like?

Abdominoplasty is performed under combined anesthesia (epidural and sedation) and usually lasts between 2 and 5 hours. The cosmetic surgeon will make a horizontal incision in the lower abdomen, similar to a cesarean section. Then, they will remove excess skin and fat, tighten the abdominal muscles, and reposition the belly button. Finally, they will close the incision with sutures.

## What is the Recovery Like?

After surgery, it's normal to have swelling, bruising, and discomfort in the abdomen. You'll need to wear a compression garment to reduce swelling and support the abdominal muscles during recovery. It's also important to avoid strenuous activities during the first few weeks. Most people can return to their normal activities in 2-4 weeks, but complete recovery can take several months.

## What are the Risks?

As with any surgery, there are risks associated with abdominoplasty. It's crucial to discuss these risks with your cosmetic surgeon before making a decision. Some of the risks include:

- **Infection:** The infection rate after a tummy tuck is generally low, but it can vary depending on factors

like the patient's health and the extent of the procedure.
- **Bleeding:** Excessive bleeding is uncommon but can occur in some cases.
- **Scarring problems:** The tummy tuck scar is usually long, and although cosmetic surgeons strive to make it as discreet as possible, scarring problems can occur in some patients.
- **Adverse reactions to anesthesia:** As with any surgical procedure, there is a small risk of adverse reactions to anesthesia.
- **Seromas:** Fluid accumulation (seroma) under the skin is a relatively common complication but can usually be managed with drainage or aspiration.
- **Skin necrosis:** In rare cases, skin necrosis (tissue death) can occur, especially in smokers or patients with certain medical conditions.
- **Deep vein thrombosis (DVT):** DVT is a serious complication that involves the formation of blood clots in the deep veins, usually in the legs. The risk of DVT after a tummy tuck is low but can increase in patients with certain risk factors.

## Frequently Asked Questions about Tummy Tucks

- **Will it hurt a lot?** Postoperative pain is usually moderate and can be controlled with medication.
- **Will I have a large scar?** The tummy tuck scar is usually long but can be hidden with underwear or a swimsuit.
- **How long do the results last?** The results of a tummy tuck can be long-lasting if you maintain a stable weight and a healthy lifestyle.

**Bibliography**

- American Society of Plastic Surgeons. (2023). Plastic Surgery Statistics Report.
- Rohrich, R. J., & Adams, W. P. Jr. (2001). Abdominoplasty: Principles and Techniques.
- Matarasso, A., & Levine, S. M. (2012). Abdominoplasty: Principles and Techniques.

# Chapter 7

# Facial and Neck Rejuvenation: Refresh Your Face!

Do you feel like your face no longer reflects the energy and vitality you have inside? Don't worry, facial and neck rejuvenation can be the solution! This set of surgical procedures can help you combat the signs of aging and regain a fresher, more youthful appearance.

### What is Facial and Neck Rejuvenation?

Facial and neck rejuvenation encompasses several surgeries that aim to improve the appearance of your face and neck. These surgeries can include facelifts (rhytidectomy), brow lifts, blepharoplasty (eyelid surgery), chin liposuction, and fat transfer.

### Am I a Good Candidate for this Type of Surgery?

If you're bothered by sagging skin, wrinkles, or excess fat on your face and neck, you could be a good candidate! But the most important thing is to have realistic expectations and understand that facial rejuvenation doesn't stop aging but helps you look better at this stage of your life. Ideally, you should be in good physical and mental health and have a clear idea of the results you expect to achieve.

### What Types of Rejuvenation are There?

There are different types of facial and neck rejuvenation, depending on your needs and goals:

- **Facelift (rhytidectomy):** Tightens facial muscles, removes excess skin, and smooths deep wrinkles.
- **Brow lift:** Lifts sagging eyebrows and reduces forehead wrinkles.
- **Blepharoplasty (eyelid surgery):** Removes excess skin and fat from the eyelids, improving the appearance of the eyes.
- **Chin liposuction:** Removes excess fat under the chin, defining the neck contour.
- **Fat transfer:** Uses your own fat to fill in areas of the face that have lost volume, such as the cheekbones or lips.

## What is the Surgery Like?

Each type of facial rejuvenation has its own surgical procedure. In general, they are performed under sedation and local anesthesia and can last several hours. The incisions are usually discreet and hidden in the scalp, behind the ears, or in the natural folds of the skin.

## What is the Recovery Like?

Recovery from facial rejuvenation varies depending on the type of surgery and the extent of the procedure. In general, you can expect:

- **Swelling and bruising:** These are normal and gradually disappear in the weeks following surgery.
- **Mild discomfort:** These can be controlled with medication.
- **Use of bandages or compression garments:** These help reduce swelling and keep the skin in its new position.

- **Avoid strenuous activities:** It's important to rest and avoid exertion during the first few weeks.

Most people can return to their normal activities in 2-4 weeks, but complete recovery can take several months.

## What are the Risks?

As with any surgery, there are risks associated with facial and neck rejuvenation. It's essential to talk to your cosmetic surgeon about all the possible risks and complications before making a decision. Some of the risks include:

- **Infection:** The infection rate after facial rejuvenation is low, usually less than 1%.
- **Bleeding:** Excessive bleeding is uncommon, occurring in less than 2% of cases.
- **Scarring problems:** Although the incisions are usually discreet, scarring problems can occur in some cases, such as hypertrophic scars or keloids.
- **Adverse reactions to anesthesia:** As with any surgical procedure, there is a small risk of adverse reactions to anesthesia, such as nausea, vomiting, or allergic reactions.
- **Damage to facial nerves:** In rare cases, temporary or permanent damage to facial nerves can occur, which can affect the movement of facial muscles. The incidence of this complication varies depending on the type of procedure and the surgeon's experience.
- **Hair loss:** There may be temporary or permanent hair loss around the incisions.
- **Facial asymmetry:** In some cases, there may be slight facial asymmetry after surgery.

- **Hematoma:** Accumulation of blood under the skin, which may require drainage. The incidence varies depending on the type of procedure and the surgeon's experience.
- **Seromas:** Accumulation of fluid under the skin, which may require drainage or aspiration.

## Frequently Asked Questions about Facial and Neck Rejuvenation

- **Will it hurt a lot?** Postoperative pain is usually moderate and can be controlled with medication.
- **Will I have visible scars?** Cosmetic surgeons strive to make discreet incisions and hide them in inconspicuous areas.
- **How long do the results last?** The results of facial rejuvenation can last several years, but natural aging will continue.
- **When can I wear makeup again?** Your surgeon will give you specific instructions, but you can usually wear makeup again after a few weeks.

## Bibliography

- American Society of Plastic Surgeons. (2023). Facelift. https://www.plasticsurgery.org/cosmetic-procedures/facelift
- American Society of Plastic Surgeons. (2023). Brow lift. https://www.plasticsurgery.org/cosmetic-procedures/brow-lift
- American Society of Plastic Surgeons. (2023). Eyelid surgery. https://www.plasticsurgery.org/cosmetic-procedures/eyelid-surgery
- Zins, J. E., & Becker, F. F. (2006). The Anatomy of the Aging Face.

- Nahai, F. (2011). The Art of Aesthetic Surgery: Principles and Techniques.
- Shiffman, M. A. (2012). Cosmetic Surgery: Art and Techniques.
- Baker, D. C. (2019). Complications in Facial Plastic Surgery.

*Facial and Neck Rejuvenation*

# Chapter 8

## Intimate Surgery: Regain Your Confidence and Well-being!

Did you know that cosmetic surgery isn't just about improving your external appearance but also your intimate well-being? Intimate surgery, also known as genital surgery or vaginal rejuvenation, can help you improve the function and appearance of your genitals, increasing your confidence and quality of life.

**What is Intimate Surgery?**

Intimate surgery encompasses several surgical procedures that aim to improve the appearance and function of female genitals. These procedures can include labiaplasty (reduction of labia minora), vaginoplasty (vaginal tightening), hymenoplasty (hymen reconstruction), and G-spot amplification.

**Am I a Good Candidate for Intimate Surgery?**

If you experience physical discomfort, discomfort during sexual intercourse, or insecurities related to the appearance of your genitals, you could be a good candidate!

**Types of Intimate Surgery**

There are different types of intimate surgery, each focused on a specific aspect:

• **Labiaplasty** (reduction of labia): Reduces the size of the labia minora when they are too large or asymmetrical.

- **Vaginoplasty** (vaginal narrowing): Narrows the vaginal canal when it has widened due to childbirth or aging.
- **Hymenoplasty** (hymen reconstruction): Reconstructs the hymen for cultural or personal reasons.
- **G-spot amplification**: Increases G-spot sensitivity to improve sexual satisfaction.

## What are the Operations Like?

Each type of intimate surgery has its own surgical procedure. In general, they are performed under local or general anesthesia and usually last between 1 and 2 hours. The incisions are usually small and hidden in the natural folds of the skin.

## What is Recovery Like?

Recovery from intimate surgery varies depending on the type of procedure. In general, you can expect:

- **Swelling and bruising**: These are normal and gradually disappear in the weeks following surgery.
- **Mild discomfort**: They can be controlled with medication.
- **Use of cold compresses**: They help reduce inflammation.
- **Avoid sexual relations**: During the first weeks, it is important to avoid sexual relations to allow proper healing.

Most women can return to normal activities within 1-2 weeks, but it is important to follow your cosmetic surgeon's instructions for optimal recovery.

## What Risks are There?

As with any surgery, there are risks associated with intimate surgery. It is crucial to discuss these risks with your cosmetic surgeon before making a decision. Some of the risks include:

- **Infection**: The infection rate after intimate surgery is generally low, but can vary depending on the type of procedure and the health of the patient.
- **Bleeding**: Excessive bleeding is rare, but can occur in some cases.
- **Healing problems**: Although the incisions are usually small, healing problems may occur in some patients, such as hypertrophic scars or keloids.
- **Adverse reactions to anesthesia**: As with any surgical procedure, there is a small risk of adverse reactions to anesthesia.
- **Loss of sensation**: In some cases, there may be a temporary or permanent decrease in sensation in the genital area.
- **Hypertrophic scars**: These are thick, raised scars that can be aesthetically unpleasant.
- **Chronic pain**: In rare cases, chronic pain may persist after surgery.

## Frequently Asked Questions about Intimate Surgery

- **Will it hurt a lot?** Postoperative pain is usually mild and can be controlled with medication.
- **Will I have visible scars?** The incisions are usually small and hidden in the natural folds of the skin.
- **How long does results last?** The results of intimate surgery can be long-lasting, but can be affected by factors such as aging and childbirth.

**Bibliography**

- American Society of Plastic Surgeons. (2023). Labiaplasty.
- American Society of Plastic Surgeons. (2023). Vaginoplasty.
- Goodman, M. P. (2013). Female Cosmetic Genital Surgery.
- Miklos, J. R., & Moore, R. D. (2018). Labiaplasty and Vaginoplasty.
- Alter, G. J. (2020). Aesthetic Vaginal Rejuvenation.
- Monstrey, S., & Selvaggi, G. (2022). Female Genital Cosmetic Surgery: A Practical Guide.

# Chapter 9

## Other Cosmetic Surgeries and Treatments: Explore your options!

Do you want to improve your appearance but are not sure which procedure is right for you? In this chapter, I present an overview of other popular cosmetic surgeries and non-surgical treatments that can help you achieve your goals.

**What other Cosmetic Surgeries are There?**

- Otoplasty (ear surgery): Corrects prominent or deformed ears.
- Mentoplasty (chin surgery): Increases or reduces the size of the chin to improve facial harmony.
- Arm lift (brachioplasty): Removes excess skin and fat from the arms.
- Thigh lift (cruroplasty): Removes excess skin and fat from the thighs.

**What Non-surgical Treatments exist?**

- Botulinum toxin (Botox): Reduces wrinkles and expression lines.
- Facial fillers: They restore lost volume and smoothen wrinkles.
- Tensor threads: Lift and make sagging skin firm.
- Chemical peels: Improve skin texture and tone.
- Lasers: Treat spots, scars and other skin problems.

**Remember!**

**Before undergoing any cosmetic surgery or treatment, it is essential that you consult with a certified and experienced cosmetic surgeon. He or she will help you evaluate your options, determine if you are a good candidate, and explain the risks and benefits of each procedure.**

**Bibliography**

- American Society of Plastic Surgeons. (2023). What is plastic surgery?
- American Board of Cosmetic Surgery. (2023). Find a cosmetic surgeon.
- Rohrich, R. J., & Pessa, J. E. (2007). The artistry of aesthetic surgery: Principles and techniques.
- Niechajev, I. (2010). Non-surgical facial rejuvenation.
- Gold, M.H. (2014). Botulinum toxin (Botox) applications in aesthetic medicine.

# Chapter 10

## Pre- and Post-Operative Care: Get Ready to Look Amazing!

You're almost ready for your transformation, but before you enter the operating room, it's important to prepare properly and know what to expect after surgery. Here's everything you need to know to make your experience as smooth and successful as possible!

**Before Surgery:**

- **Medical consultation:** First things first: a complete medical checkup! Your cosmetic surgeon will assess you to ensure you're in good health and suitable for surgery.
- **Preoperative studies:** You'll be asked for some laboratory tests, such as blood tests and an electrocardiogram, to rule out any health problems that could interfere with the surgery.
- **Quit smoking:** If you smoke, it's time to say goodbye to cigarettes. Smoking affects healing and increases the risk of complications, so quit at least a few weeks before and after surgery.
- **Avoid certain medications:** Some medications, such as aspirin and anticoagulants, can increase the risk of bleeding. Your surgeon will tell you which ones you should stop taking before surgery.
- **Plan your recovery:** Make sure you have everything ready at home for your recovery, such as medications, easy-to-prepare food, comfortable clothes, and someone to help you with daily tasks.

**After Surgery:**

- **Rest:** Give your body time to recover. Get enough rest and avoid strenuous activities during the first few weeks.
- **Medications:** Take the medications prescribed by your surgeon to control pain, inflammation, and prevent infections.
- **Wound care:** Keep the wounds clean and dry according to your surgeon's instructions.
- **Compression garments:** You may need to wear compression garments to reduce swelling and help the skin adapt to its new shape.
- **Follow-up appointments:** Attend all your follow-up appointments with your surgeon so they can assess your progress and ensure you're recovering properly.

**Don't Worry!**

It's normal to feel some anxiety before surgery, but remember that you're in good hands. As a personal recommendation, you must visualize the outcome, not to put high hopes but to put your mind in the proper mindset, your brain does not know whether you are anxious or excited, so remind yourself that you are super excited, instead of releasing cortisol, you will be releasing endorphins and your body and recovery will appreciate it. Your cosmetic surgeon will guide you through every step of the process and provide you with all the information you need to feel safe and calm.

**And remember...**

Cosmetic surgery is a tool to improve your appearance and self-esteem, but it's not a substitute for a healthy life. Maintain a balanced diet, exercise regularly, and take care of your skin to prolong the results of your surgery and feel good inside and out.

I hope this guide has been helpful and has helped you clear up your doubts about cosmetic surgery. Remember that the decision to undergo a cosmetic procedure is personal and should be made calmly and after being well-informed. If you have any other questions or need more information, do not hesitate to consult with a certified plastic surgeon. He or she will be happy to help you achieve your aesthetic goals and help you feel more confident and happy with yourself to reflect your inner beauty to the outside world.

# About the Author

Dr. Daniel Gallaga was a Professor of Anatomy at the Autonomous University of Baja California (UABC). He has a Certification in Stem Cells and is an Active Member of the American Academy of Cosmetic Surgery.

He is an expert in the following: Eyelid Lift, with brow lift single incision; High-definition Tummy Tuck; Breast Augmentation (no bra, no touch personal technique); Breast Lift; Laser integrated Face Lift; Laser Chin Liposuction; and Ultrasound-guided Brazilian Butt Lift (BBL) for patient safety.

In addition, he has been a Medical Specialist in Aesthetic Surgery in various prestigious institutions such as Vive Medical Spa, Skinklinik, CEDApiel, among others. He is a Founding Partner of Cosmetic Clinic.

Currently, Dr. Gallaga works at the Cosmetic Clinic and continues his academic career to deliver the most novel techniques for his patients.

www.ingramcontent.com/pod-product-compliance
Lightning Source LLC
Chambersburg PA
CBHW030512220526
45464CB00006B/2757